INTERMITTENT FASTING FOR WOMEN OVER 50

THE ESSENTIAL GUIDE TO INCREASING ENERGY, BURNING FAT, AND RESETTING METABOLISM. SLOW THE AGING PROCESS AND DETOX YOUR BODY THANKS TO INTERMITTENT FASTING

Table of Contents

Introduction

Once we age beyond 50 years, our bodies start to change in the ways they handle certain things. Sugar, fat, and diets as a whole. You might find that things you could eat with no issue as recently as five years ago are suddenly giving you heartburn or causing you to have troubles when it's time to go to the restroom. For many of these, it strikes us as a cruel aspect of reality, and it seems like we're moving past the things that we enjoy in life and that we're relegated to less interesting meals.

While this is a negative frame of mind, I completely understand it, and you're entitled to feel that way at first. It is important to know, however, that your metabolism and your body are simply shifting into a different phase and that you've got a lot of other things going on, especially hormone-wise. You will find that things like menopause and certain other aspects of the aging process are the reasons we have to adjust a lot of things. You might be surprised to learn that the things you eat do have a bearing on how you're feeling, and they do have a bearing on how quickly and easily your body adapts to those changes. I'm not saying they're solely responsible, simply that the fuel you're giving your body does make a difference.

With intermittent fasting, your focus is not only on the structure you use for your meal consumption but also on ensuring that your body is getting all of the whole nutrients it needs in order to function properly while you're eating. If you commit to doing the intermittent fasting regimen, you must also commit to making sure that your meals contain all the right things to sustain you, to activate the right hormone production in your body, and the supplemental nutrition you will need in order to make the very most of the time your body is spending breaking down the fat stores in your body for crucial nutrition and energy.

While your body is making these adjustments in the way, it's continuing to regenerate cells for hair, skin, organs, etc., it is making use of the food you're giving it in order to do those things. If you're able to provide your body with the ideal balance of macronutrients (fat, protein, and carbohydrates) from ideal and nourishing sources, you will find that your body simply thrives on what it's been given. You will find that the processes in your body, everything from the simple stuff like sleeping to the more complex stuff like organ health, will continue on with more ease.

Some women in this age group have found themselves grappling with things that were never a problem for them before. Some women find that in spite of the fact that they were carrying on through their days while feeling like they could fall asleep standing up and any moment, they are completely unable to sleep when the time finally comes for them to hang up their hats for the day. Some women find that around the time they would typically be menstruating, their bodies are throwing curveballs at them that are simply impossible to anticipate. Some women find that their digestive system simply won't process things in the way that it once did.

Our bodies tend to need a much higher balance of things like vitamins, minerals, fiber, and things that can tend to be forgotten in the everyday diet unless you've spent a lot of time being very health-conscious. Many of us have simply been busy living our lives, minding what we eat, exercising when we can, without breaking down the daily values and percentages of everything we eat to find out what works best. Most of us haven't conducted our diets using the scientific method, figuring out what measures of certain nutrients are better than others.

While intermittent fasting doesn't go that far, it can certainly feel like that in the beginning, and it is crucial that you be on the lookout for the changes in your body and your overall wellness to ensure that you're making changes for the better and that your body is gaining benefits from the methods and foods you're using from day to day.

For women of our age, it can seem like there are just a lot of things going on in our bodies all at once, and you really wouldn't be wrong in assuming that. Where you might be mistaken in your assumption, however, is that it doesn't need to be the end of the world, and it doesn't have to be very hard to turn the ship around. You have a lot of life ahead of you, and you have a lot left to do here with life, family, goals, and all the things you have worked so hard for in your life.

Life is meant to be enjoyed, and that does not change, no matter what age you've reached. Intermittent fasting is here to give you the tools to make life enjoyable, so you can continue to do what makes life worth living without having to suffer at the hands of changing bodily processes and hormone outputs!

Chapter 1 . Differences in Metabolism Between a Young Woman and a Healthy Over 50

At the most basic level, it must be said that there are detailed bodily differences between young women and older women. Many of these bodily differences become obvious with the outward, physical effects of aging, but a lot of them also happen on the inside, away from what our eyes can see.

When women age, enter and exit menopause, and become fully mature, their bodies change, reflecting different nutritional needs for the next 30+ years. During menopause, in particular, certain foods help with the urges, hot flashes, and more, but the period of intense transition is more of a gateway into a completely altered future (mentally, bodily, nutritionally, and more).

Women of this age experience slowed metabolism (to their great frustrations) as well as lowered hormone production. For weight and mood, therefore, menopause and maturation are equal disasters. Your body will go completely "out of whack," compared to how it used to function. You'll likely put on weight despite the dietary choices you make, and you may feel there's no relief in sight. Don't be fooled, however! Things may have changed for you, but they won't be stagnant changes.

Essentially, women at the stage of menopause and beyond need to absorb less energy overall from their food, yet they need more protein to deal with the effects of aging. Vitamins B12 & D, calcium, and zinc will need to be boosted, while iron becomes less important for the aging female body. Vitamins C, E, A, & beta-carotene need to be increased too in order to fight off cancer, infection, disease, and more.

As the woman ages and matures even further, more things will change; mainly, she cannot bypass taking these important supplements any longer. In older and more mature women, the body's abilities to recognize hunger and thirst become muted, and dehydration poses a greater threat. Fewer calories are required for the older and more mature woman too, but she still needs to get as many nutrients as (if not more than!) the young woman does.

It seems that a younger woman can eat (relatively) what she wants and not worry about taking vitamins or supplements, but it is undeniable that the older woman will need this nutritional help to ensure longevity. Basically, health needs become more pressing for women at this age, as their bodies are less flexible and resistant to problems that may arise.

How IF Affects Women at This Age & How to Approach It

Because health, diet, reproductivity, and nutritional needs are all altered for mature and menopausal women, their relationships with intermittent fasting can be very different from young women. For instance, while young women ought to be careful about how intermittent fasting can affect their fertility levels, older women can practice intermittent fasting freely without these concerns. Therefore, more mature women can apply the weight-loss techniques of intermittent fasting to their lives (and waistlines) without the worry of what negative side-effects might arise in the future.

For menopausal women, however, the situation is a little bit different than it is for fully mature women. People going through menopause have to deal with daily hormone fluctuations that cause hot and cold flashes, sleeplessness, anxiety, irregular periods, and more. At the beginning of this process, intermittent fasting will not necessarily help, and it could even make your situation more stressful.

For women in this situation who are actively going through menopause, you must remember that your body is extremely sensitive to changes right now. If you do find that intermittent fasting helps and that short periods of fast are effective, you must also make sure to increase the intensity of your fast as gradually as possible so your body can adjust without creating horrible hormonal repercussions for yourself and everyone around you. For the fully mature woman, intermittent fasting will not make you as cranky, moody, irregular in the period, or otherwise because those hormones won't be affecting you at all anymore, or at least, hardly at all. Your dietary and eating schedule choices become more liberated from the effects they used to have on your hormonal health as the years go by. Therefore, if you're seeking weight loss, better energy, a physiological jolt back to health, or what have you, try out IF without concern and see what happens. For these types of women, intermittent fasting is set to provide hope through eased depression, the lessened likelihood of cancer (or its recurrence), promised weight loss, and more.

Chapter 2 . Advantages and Disadvantages of Fasting

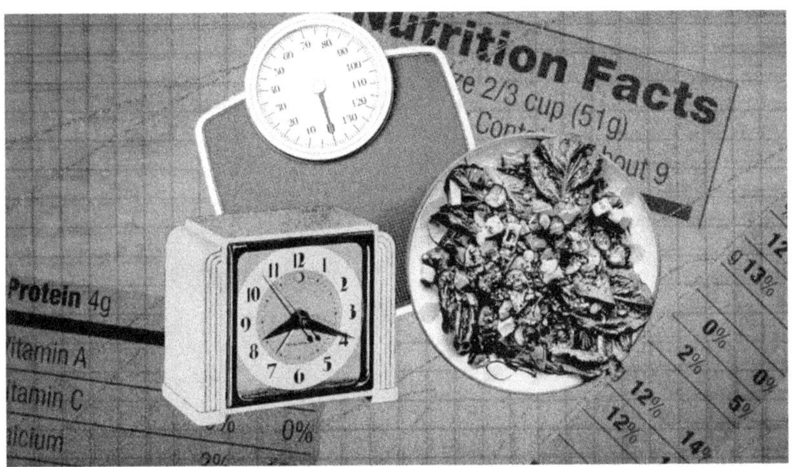

The different dietary examples have gotten consideration as an approach to reach and keep up a solid weight and to pick up wellbeing benefits even on ineffectively sound people.

Research is progressing to completely comprehend the upsides and downsides of intermittent fasting. Long haul contemplates are missing to know without a doubt if this eating style gives enduring advantages:

Pros

Simple to Follow

Numerous dietary examples center around eating specific nourishments and restricting or keeping away from different food sources. Learning the particular standards of an eating style can require a significant time duty. For instance, there are whole books committed to understanding the DASH diet or figuring out how to follow a Mediterranean-style feast plan. On an eating plan that joins Intermittent fasting, you just eat as indicated by the hour of day or day of the week. When you've figured out which intermittent fasting convention is best for you, all you need is a watch or a schedule to realize when to eat.

No Calorie Counting

As anyone might expect, individuals who are attempting to reach or keep up a sound weight for the most part like to maintain a strategic distance from calorie tallying. While nutrition names are effectively found on numerous nourishments, the way toward estimating segment measures and organizing day-by-day tallies either physically or on a cell phone application can be dull.

An investigation distributed in 2011 found that individuals are bound to follow plans when all pre-estimated calorie-controlled nourishments are provided. Commercial eating diets, for example, WW, Jenny Craig, and others offer these types of assistance for a charge. Nonetheless, numerous individuals don't have the assets to pay for these kinds of projects, particularly in the long haul. Intermittent fasting gives a basic elective where practically no calorie-checking is required. Much of the time, calorie limitation (and along these lines, weight loss) happens in light of the fact that nourishment is either wiped out or essentially confined on specific days or during specific hours of the day.

No Macronutrient Limitations

There are well-known eating plans that essentially confine explicit macronutrients. For instance, numerous individuals who follow low-carb eating intend to support wellbeing or get in shape. Others follow a low-fat eating diet for restorative or weight loss purposes. Every one of these projects requires the shopper to embrace another method for eating, regularly supplanting most loved nourishments with new and perhaps new food sources. This may require new cooking abilities and figuring out how to shop and stock the kitchen in an unexpected way.

None of these abilities are required when intermittent fasting is basically on the grounds that there is no objective macronutrient extend and no macronutrient is limited or taboo.

Unrestricted Eating

Any individual who has ever changed their eating routine to accomplish a health advantage or arrive at a solid weight realizes that you begin to desire nourishments that you are advised not to eat. Indeed, an investigation distributed in 2017 affirmed that an expanded drive to eat is a key factor during a weight loss venture.

In any case, this test is explicitly constrained on an Intermittent Fasting plan. Nourishment limitation just happens during certain restricted hours, and on the non-fasting hours or days of the arrangement, you can, by and large, eat anything you desire. Truth be told, specialists here and there call nowadays "devouring" days.

Obviously, proceeding to eat undesirable nourishments may not be the most advantageous approach to pick up profits by Intermittent fasting; however, removing them during specific days constrains your general intake and may at last give benefits.

Might Boost Longevity

One of the most broadly referred advantages of intermittent fasting includes life span. As indicated by the National Institute on Aging, rat examines have demonstrated that when mice are put on projects that seriously confine calories (regularly during fasting periods), many demonstrated an augmentation of life expectancy and diminished paces of a few ailments, particularly malignant growths.

So, does this advantage reach out to people? As per the individuals who advance the eating diets, it does. Nonetheless, long-haul contemplates are expected to affirm the advantage. As indicated by a survey distributed in 2010, there have been observational researches connecting strict fasting to long-haul life span benefits, yet it was difficult to decide whether fasting gave the advantage or whenever related variables had an impact.

Advances Weight Loss

In a survey of intermittent fasting research distributed in 2018, creators report that the examinations they inspected indicated a huge diminishing in fat mass among subjects who took an interest in clinical preliminaries. They additionally saw that intermittent fasting was found as productive in decreasing weight, regardless of the weight list. It is conceivable, in any case, that IF is not any more powerful than conventional calorie limitation. Intermittent fasting might not be any more compelling than different weight control plans that confine calories all the time. A recent report contrasted intermittent fasting and customary eating diets (characterized as constant energy limitation) and found that weight loss benefits are comparable. It is likewise conceivable that weight loss results may rely upon age. An examination distributed in the diary

Nutrition in 2018 inspected the impacts of intermittent fasting (time-limited benefiting from) youthful (20-year-old) versus more established (50-year-elderly people) men. Intermittent fasting somewhat diminished weight in the youthful, however not in the more established men. Nonetheless, muscle power remained the equivalent in the two gatherings.

Glucose Control

In 2018, some intermittent fasting specialists recommended that this eating style may help those with type 2 diabetes oversee glucose. In any case, the discoveries have been conflicting.

Nonetheless, another investigation distributed in 2019 indicated a less amazing effect on blood glucose control. Scientists led a two-year follow-up of a year mediation contrasting intermittent fasting and persistent calorie limitation in individuals with type 2 diabetes. They found that HbA1c levels expanded in both the constant calorie limitation and intermittent gatherings at 2 years. These discoveries were reliable with results from different investigations demonstrating that notwithstanding the scope of dietary mediations it isn't unprecedented for blood glucose levels to increment after some time in those with type 2 diabetes. The examination creators do note, notwithstanding, that Intermittent energy limitation might be better than ceaseless energy limitation for keeping up lower HbA1c levels, yet noticed that more investigations are expected to affirm the advantage.

Proven Health Benefits

IF is an eating practice in which you switch between eating and fasting times. Intermittent fasting can be achieved in a variety of ways, like the 16/8 or 5:2 routines. Numerous studies have shown it can have important health and cognitive benefits. Here are ten health advantages of intermittent fasting that have been scientifically proven.

1. **Intermittent Fasting Changes the Function of Cells, Genes, and Hormones**

When you don't eat for a while, your body goes through a number of changes.

To make stored body fat more available, your body, for example, initiates essential cellular repair processes and adjusts hormone levels.

Here are some of the physiological changes that happen during fasting:

- **Insulin levels:** Insulin levels in the blood drop dramatically, promoting fat burning.

- **Human growth hormone:** Growth hormone levels in the blood will rise by up to 5-fold. Increased levels of this hormone aid with fat loss and muscle growth, among other things.

- **Cellular repair:** The body initiates essential cellular repair procedures, such as the removal of waste from cells.

- **Gene expression:** There are beneficial variations in various genes and molecules connected to survival and disease prevention.

These variations in hormones, gene expression, and cell function are linked to several of the advantages of intermittent fasting.

Insulin levels fall, and human growth hormone levels rise when you fast. Your cells also initiate critical cellular repair processes and alter the expression of genes.

2. Intermittent Fasting Can Help You Lose Weight and Belly Fat

Many people who experiment with intermittent fasting do so in terms of weight loss. In general, intermittent fasting causes you to eat fewer meals. You will consume fewer calories unless you compensate by consuming even more often during the other meals.

Intermittent fasting also improves hormone function, which aids weight loss. Reduced insulin levels, greater growth hormone levels, and higher norepinephrine levels all help the body break down fat and use it for energy.

As a result, short-term fasting boosts metabolic rate by 3.7–14%, allowing you to eat even more calories. Intermittent fasting, in other words, operates on both ends of the calorie equation. It increases your metabolic rate (calories expended) while decreasing the quantity of food you consume (reduces calories).

According to the scientific literature 2014 review, intermittent fasting results in a weight loss of 3 to 8% over 3 to 24 weeks. This is a huge number. The participants also lost 4 to 7% of the waist circumference, showing they lost an excess of belly fat, the disease-causing fat in the abdominal cavity.

3. **Intermittent fasting will lower the risk of Type 2 diabetes by reducing insulin resistance.**

In recent decades, type 2 diabetes is becoming extremely popular. The high blood sugar level in the sense of insulin resistance is the most prominent characteristic. Anything that decreases insulin resistance and protects against type 2 diabetes should decrease blood sugar levels.

Intermittent fasting is said to have tangible advantages for insulin resistance and to result in a significant drop in blood sugar levels. Intermittent fasting has been shown to lower fasting blood sugar by 3–6% and fasting insulin by 20–31% in human studies.

Intermittent fasting also prevented diabetic rats from kidney injury, which is one of the most serious complications of diabetes. This means that intermittent fasting could be very beneficial for people at risk for type 2 diabetes.

There might, however, be some gender differences. According to a study, after a 22-day intermittent fasting regimen, blood sugar control in women worsened. At least in men, intermittent fasting can lower insulin resistance and lower blood sugar levels.

4. Intermittent fasting can help the body decrease oxidative stress and inflammation.

One of the steps toward aging and many chronic diseases is oxidative stress. It includes unstable molecules known as free radicals interacting with and destroying other essential molecules (such as protein and DNA). Intermittent fasting has been shown in many studies to improve the body's resistance to oxidative stress.

In addition, studies show that intermittent fasting can help tackle inflammation, which is a major cause of a variety of diseases. This should help prevent aging and the onset of a variety of diseases.

5. Intermittent fasting may be good for your heart.

Heart disease is still the world's leading cause of death. Various health indicators (also known as "risk factors") have been linked to a decreased or increased risk of heart disease.

Intermittent fasting has been shown to increase blood pressure, inflammatory markers, blood triglycerides, blood sugar levels, and total and LDL cholesterol, among other risk factors.

However, a significant portion of this is focused on animal research. Before any recommendations can be made, further research on the impact on humans' heart health is needed.

6. Intermittent fasting activates several cellular repair mechanisms.

When we fast, our bodies' cells start a process called autophagy, which is a cellular "waste removal" process. Broken and damaged proteins that accumulate within cells over time are broken down and metabolized by the cells. Increased autophagy can protect against cancer and Alzheimer's disease, among other diseases

7. Intermittent fasting can aid in cancer prevention.

Cancer is a horrific disease that is characterized by uncontrollable cell development. Fasting has also been shown to have a number of metabolic benefits, including a lower risk of cancer.

Despite the lack of human studies, promising evidence from animal studies suggests that intermittent fasting may help to hinder cancer. Fasting minimized multiple side effects of chemotherapy in human cancer patients, according to some evidence.

8. Intermittent fasting is beneficial to your mental health.

What is beneficial for health is frequently also good for the brain. Intermittent fasting increases a variety of metabolic characteristics that are related to brain health.

Reduced oxidative stress, blood sugar levels, inflammation, and insulin resistance are all part of this. Intermittent fasting has been shown in many experiments in rats to increase the development of new nerve cells, which could boost brain function.

It also raises levels of a brain hormone known as a brain-derived neurotrophic factor (BDNF), whose deficiency has been related to depression and other neurological issues. Intermittent fasting has also been shown to protect against brain damage caused by strokes in animals.

9. Intermittent fasting can reduce the risk of Alzheimer's disease.

The most prominent neurodegenerative disease in the world is Alzheimer's disease. Since there is no cure for Alzheimer's disease, stopping it from occurring in the first place is important. According to a rat study, intermittent fasting can delay the onset of Alzheimer's disease or minimize its severity.

According to a series of case reports, a lifestyle modification that included regular short-term fasts was able to substantially boost

Alzheimer's symptoms in 9 out of 10 patients. According to animal studies, fasting may also defend against other neurodegenerative disorders, such as Parkinson's and Huntington's disease. However, further human research is needed.

10. Intermittent fasting can help you live longer by extending your life span.

One of the most intriguing benefits of intermittent fasting is the potential to prolong life span. Intermittent fasting increases lifespan in rats in the same way as constant calorie restriction does. The results of a few of these experiments were very dramatic. One of them found that rats who fasted every other day survived 83 % longer than rats who didn't fast.

Intermittent fasting has become very common among the anti-aging crowd, even though it has yet to be demonstrated in humans. Given the benefits of intermittent fasting for metabolism and various health indicators, it's easy to see how it could assist you in living a healthier and longer life.

Cons

Side Effects

Studies exploring the advantages of Intermittent fasting additionally point to certain symptoms that may happen during the fasting phase of the eating program.

For instance, it isn't remarkable to feel grouchy, tired, and experience cerebral pains when your calories are seriously limited. Almost certainly, these reactions will happen when nourishment is altogether dispensed with (for instance, during programs like substitute day fasting) and more averse to happen when nourishment intake is diminished, (for example, on the 5:2 eating diet when 500–600 calories are devoured during fasting days).

Decreased Physical Activity

One eminent reaction of intermittent fasting might be the decrease in physical activity. Most Intermittent fasting programs do exclude a suggestion for physical movement. Of course, the individuals who follow the projects may encounter enough exhaustion that they neglect to meet everyday step objectives and may even change their ordinary exercise schedules.

Proceeding with inquiring about has been proposed to perceive how intermittent fasting may influence physical action designs.

Extreme Hunger

As anyone might expect, it is regular for those in the fasting phase of an IF eating intends to encounter serious appetite. This craving may turn out to be increasingly outrageous when they are around other people who are devouring common dinners and bites.

Medications

Numerous individuals who take meds locate that taking their solution with nourishment assists with certain soothing symptoms. Truth be told, a few meds explicitly convey the proposal that they ought to be taken with nourishment. Hence, taking meds during fasting might be a test.

Any individual who takes drugs ought to address their medicinal services supplier before beginning an IF convention to be certain that the fasting stage won't meddle with the prescription's viability or symptoms.

No Focus on Nutritious Eating

The foundation of most intermittent fasting programs is timing, instead of nourishment decision. Along these lines, no nourishments (counting those that need great nutrition) are stayed away from, and nourishments that give great nutrition are not advanced. Hence, those following the eating diet don't really figure out how to eat a solid eating diet.

May Promote Overeating

During the "devouring" phase of numerous intermittent fasting conventions, feast size and supper recurrence are not limited. Rather, shoppers appreciate a not indispensable eating diet. Sadly, this may advance indulging in certain individuals. For instance, if you feel denied following a day of complete fasting, you may feel slanted to indulge (or eat inappropriate nourishments) on days when "devouring" is permitted

Long-term Limitations

While the act of intermittent fasting isn't new, a great part of the examination exploring the advantages of this eating style is moderately later. Consequently, it is difficult to discern whether the advantages are durable. Furthermore, specialists regularly remark that long-haul considers are expected to decide whether the eating plan is even safe for over a while.

Until further notice, the most secure strategy is to work with your human services supplier when picking and beginning an IF program. Your social insurance group can screen your advancement, including medical advantages and worries, to ensure that the eating style is solid for you.

Who Shouldn't Fast Intermittently?

Although intermittent fasting is healthy, it is not a form of diet that we can all use. First and foremost, please speak to an advisor regarding intermittent fasting, particularly if you have identified medical problems before beginning your routine. If you're unclear whether intermittent fasting is appropriate for you, this list might point out explanations for maybe not doing it.

People with Eating Disorders

If you have an eating disorder or previously had an eating disorder, it could be safer to stop intermittent fasting. Anyone with eating disorders may have an obsessiveness with dieting, and it may be attributed to psychological factors and not anything that is physiologically wrong with you.

Diabetics

While intermittent fasting decreases insulin and can be helpful to those who avoid diabetes, in certain situations, it may not be a successful approach. If you do have diabetes, it's better to speak to the doctor because the variations in type 1 diabetes and type 2 diabetes in your particular case may mean that you don't have the correct intermittent fasting.

Serious Fitness Fanatics and Athletes

What if you're committed to a rigorous workout schedule already? Intermittent fasting will help you, and it can potentially hinder your success too. Athletes require calories, and their bodies are now functioning to lose fat and to strengthen their muscles. This intensity enables nutrition to be a huge factor in their success; through rest and good eating, they seek to cure their bodies, looking at their nutrients, not just calories. Athletes seem to use more calories, of course, than the normal individual who is not as active. Although intermittent fasting is achievable on a strict exercise schedule, proper planning is necessary to ensure that the body isn't overworking.

People Who Have Issues with Digestion

As if digestive problems were not too complicated to contend with on their own, introducing a wonky eating routine to the equation will just create further gastrointestinal discomfort. "If you have digestive issues (e.g., IBS), intermittent fasting can worsen the symptoms, or may even intensify digestive problems due to extended fasting bouts." Fasting cycles can interrupt the usual digestive system function, causing constipation, indigestion, and bloating. Gastrointestinal discomfort may be induced by consuming large meals, sometimes needed for IF forms that call for long-term fasting. "This is especially troubling for those with IBS who also have a more sensitive gut.

Nutrition, Concentration, and Motivation Are Critical to Everyday Activities

Food gives sustenance and strength that helps you to concentrate. When you're incredibly hungry, what you can think about is food that distracts the mind from the actual tasks at hand. If you have the sort of job or are involved in sports where strength and focus are required, intermittent fasting might not be appropriate for you.

Pregnant or Breastfeeding Women

Involving in it during pregnancy or breastfeeding may pose a risk to a child's health.

Pregnancy and breastfeeding need sufficient calorie consumption for the proper development of the baby and milk productivity. Fasting cycles will mess with your food consumption, so breastfeeding and pregnant women shouldn't do intermittent fasting. "If you're attempting to get pregnant, IF may not be the diet of preference for you either. IF can even be related to fertility problems, triggering menstrual shifts, metabolic disturbances, and even early menopause in women.

People on Medications That Have to Be Taken with Food

These are several medicines that need to be consumed in the presence of food because without it, among many other side effects, they can render you feel nauseated or light-headed. Also, individuals who take a number of vitamins or nutrients per day may be impacted by IF fasting periods. For example, people who have a low blood iron count or anemia may need to take a daily iron supplement (or several) to help recover iron levels. Iron supplements are known for inducing diarrhea and can help alleviate the sensation when consuming it with meals. The moment you take an iron supplement can be adjustable, but what if you are on a medication that needs to be administered with food and at a very particular time of the day? That's where things get a bit messy because, in the end, getting into this diet is probably not a smart choice if it doesn't fit the medications.

Those with A Weak Immune System or Have Cancer

Anyone that has undergone a significant illness previously, or is actually battling one, does not indulge in IF after first talking things up with a specialist. Here's why: "In most situations, sufficient calorie consumption is required to sustain lean body mass and a stable immune system that is vital for people with cancer or compromised immune systems," All people will speak to a specialist before trying intermittent fasting.

The Lifestyle Cannot Tolerate the Hours You Eat

Your job life will have a major effect on the willingness to participate in IF effectively. For instance, if you work the night shift and have to sleep in the afternoon because one of your feeding cycles comes in the afternoon, what do you do? Or worst, what if any of the fast happens when you are busy at work. Or, what if you work each day in various shifts and never have a regular schedule? Fasting cycles can trigger you to feel cold, with headaches and mood fluctuations. Having to deal with all those possible side effects could distract you from work and render you less efficient.

Chapter 3. Ways of Organizing Fasting According to the Rhythms of One's Life

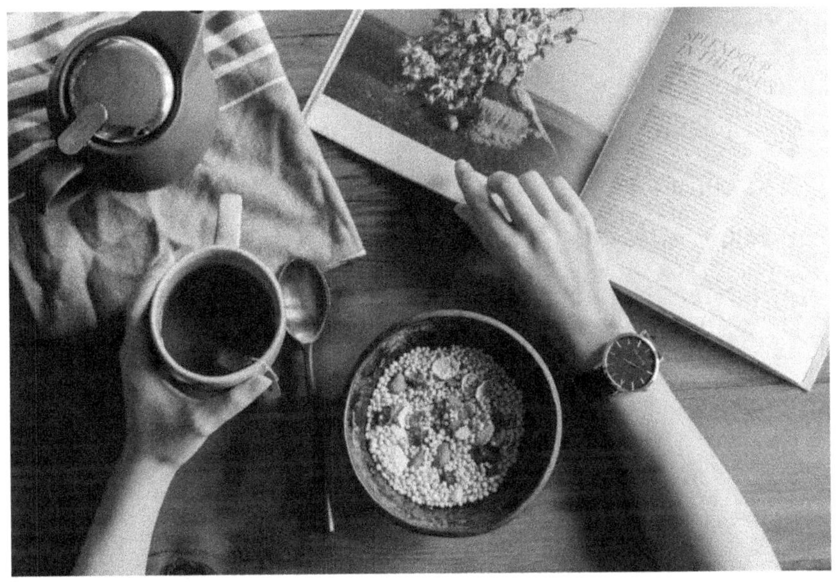

When you choose from the different options listed above, there are several things you'll want to keep in mind. First and foremost, among those things will be the fact that you can always choose another method (or a more flexible one to start with) if something doesn't work as you'd hoped.

Ultimately, you'll want to keep the following points in mind as you go about selecting your method: body type & abilities, lifestyle, daily tendencies, work routine, friends & family, and dietary choices. For all these considerations, remember what feels best to you, and remember to keep your goals with IF in mind at all times!

Consider your body type and abilities.

Think of how your body looks and feels and how much about it you'd like to change. Think about how you react to food and what it looks like when you're hungry. Think about those things you view as your "limits" and how comfortable you are with pushing. Are you a fitness freak or a couch potato? Are you huskier or slimmer? Does your body hold onto fat or build muscle quickly? Do you retain water weight or not? Do you work out? Do you require a lot of water when you do? Consider all these things about your body and more, then compare them to the methods listed above.

Consider your lifestyle.

When do you normally wake up, and how much sleep do you get on an average night? How hungry are you normally when you do wake up? How fast is your metabolism, and when do you notice its peak? How do you make your living? Do you spend a lot of time in the car or on your feet, or in an office? Are you constantly around other people, or are you often alone? When you choose your method for Intermittent Fasting, make sure to consider all these lifestyle points. Maybe you wouldn't want to choose to time with a method that disallows you to eat when you normally need the most energy. Maybe you wouldn't want to choose a method that forces you to eat when you're supposed to be at work.

Consider your daily tendencies.

Do you eat mostly in the daylight hours or after the sun goes down? Do you go to work in the daytime or nighttime? Are you generally nocturnal, diurnal, or crepuscular? Do you have a lot of freedom and flexibility in your daily routines? Do you travel a lot for work? Do you spend a lot of time on the move? Do you have trouble remembering to eat? Are you the type of person that works out on the regular? Consider these themes in your life and more before you choose your method. Does it make sense for you to have low intake days where you consume 500 calories or less? Or does it make more sense for you to have extended periods in each day where you're just not eating based on your habits or tendencies or otherwise? Plan something that makes sense and respects your habits so that the transition into Intermittent Fasting is as easy and painless as possible.

Consider your work routine.

Do you go to work in the morning or night? Are you allowed to eat at work? Do you work around food or in the food-service industry? Do you work on the feet of yours throughout the day or perhaps by doing something strenuous? Do you receive accidental or purposeful exercise opportunities at work, or perhaps are you just sitting in the same position all day? All of these elements of your work regime will be important to consider as you decide which avenue of Intermittent Fasting to go down. You won't want to engage in a method like 20:4 if you're at work every day for incredibly short shifts. 20:4 works better for someone who works very long and distracting days. You won't want to try a method like 12:12 if part of your eating window involves being at work when you're not allowed to eat at work. Remember to take your work life, routines, and restrictions into account when you go about making this choice, for you will make things much less harsh on yourself if you can look at this bigger picture from the beginning and planning stages.

Consider your friends, coworkers, and family.

How loud are their opinions? Are their lives oriented toward health? Do they demean you a lot or make fun of your choices? Or are they encouraging all the time? Are these people your support system, or are they your devils' advocates? Do you have the sense that they want to see you succeed? On the most basic level, are they nice to you and respectful of your choices? It may not seem that important, but supportive capacity and the attitudes of your family, coworkers, and friends can mean the world when you make a huge choice like starting Intermittent Fasting in your life. Occasionally, folks simply do not wish to see us succeed. They block our successes with jealousy, pride, ignorance, or arrogance. When friends and family act like this, it's better to choose a method that allows you to avoid discussing IF around them whatsoever. When friends and family are open and supportive, they shouldn't influence your choice that much; it's just when things are tenuous that you'll need to keep them (and your time around them) in consideration.

Consider your dietary choices.

Do you eat a lot of processed foods? Or do you eat a largely whole-foods, plant-based diet? Do you count calories? Do you cautiously skim nutrition facts? Are you looking for something specific like high fat, high fiber, or high protein? Are you hoping to change your diet entirely, or are you trying to keep things the way they are? Are you willing to sacrifice items of your diet to actualize your goals? All these questions help determine which type of method you're going to be ready for. Essentially, if you're trying to change your diet entirely, a method with days "on" and days "off" will work best for you. In this case, try 5:2, alternate-day, eat-stop-eat, and spontaneous skip methods. However, if you don't want to change your diet that much at all, a method where you fast for periods within each day will be desirable instead. Try methods like 20:4, 16:8, 14:10, or 12:12 for this type of situation.

As long as you make your selection with these points in mind, you're sure to succeed with your Intermittent Fasting goals. You enable yourself to make the safest, smartest, best choice for your circumstances, and that's an incredible tool to use in so many different applications. In this case, it's a tool that will help keep you healthy, boost your brain, heal your heart, and shed that excess weight like melted butter!

Chapter 4. The Importance of a Varied Diet

Intermittent Fasting on Keto Diet

Intermittent fasting and the ketogenic diet are often combined to produce stunning fat loss results. The thing about both ways of eating is that they restrict food in such a way that they promote ketosis or fat burning. They both offer similar health benefits, as well. If used together, they can result in significant fat loss.

How to Combine the Two

Combining keto and fasting is easy. The two methods of eating can work in harmony, turning your body into a sleek fat-burning machine. You pick a fasting plan that works for you, and then you eat keto-friendly foods on your eating days or during your eating windows.

Possibly the best fasting plan while on keto is the 16:8 method, or the 5:2 method. You don't need to go on long fasts while also on keto since your body is already in ketosis from the keto diet plan.

You can use intermittent fasting to reach ketosis first before launching a keto diet. Cleanse your body on a fast, such as the Warrior Method.

When you stop fasting, make sure your meals are ketogenic. You want your first meal to have lots of fat and then continue eating that way. Satiate cravings and prevent overeating during eating windows with low-carb snacks, such as almonds or carrots. Then work fasting into a cycle, balanced with days of keto eating. If you ever slip up on keto by eating too many carbs and leaving ketosis, you can get back into it by fasting for a few days again.

Before you begin this combination, find a keto calculator online for free and enter the appropriate information. You will learn how many carbohydrates, fats, proteins, and overall calories you need per day. You also want to factor in dietary fiber, which keto often neglects to mention. Most people should aim for 25–30 grams of fiber per day. Fiber is essential for your health and smooth, easy stools, which can become too fluid with the high-fat content of ketogenic foods. Fiber has carbs, but they are generally negligible and will not add to your carb allotment.

Once you know this information, you can plan meals that get you the proper amount of nutrients of each kind during your eating windows. You can use fasting time to plan these meals and prepare for them, keeping yourself busy. Just don't fall into the temptation of eating while you cook!

Benefits of the Keto Diet When You're Fasting

The main benefit of fasting on the keto diet is that you will accelerate results because you will enter ketosis faster. On the keto diet, you restrict carbs and focus on eating high-fat foods to make your body stop relying on sugar and burn fat instead. The presence of ketones in the blood or urine announces that ketosis has commenced. But it can take days and very stringent dietary control to enter ketosis on the keto diet. Since IF can trigger ketosis in a matter of days, versus weeks on ketosis, it allows for entering fat-burning mode more efficiently.

Plus, many people will find themselves out of ketosis if they slip even a tiny bit on their keto diet. A few too many blueberries or a single piece of toast can end ketosis, and then the person must start all over again to get back into it. Fasting when you slip up on keto can help you slide into ketosis again more rapidly.

The diet is simplified with a routine set by fasting, as well. You know exactly what you can eat and when. During your eating window, you should get your calculated rate of fat and protein macros and keep carbs under 20 grams per day. During fasting, you don't have to worry about what to eat at all. And yes, water and bone broth are highly useful on both keto and fasting so that you can use them throughout your diet.

The keto diet can be hard to sustain, especially if you love your pasta or donuts. So, since fasting is a way of eating that can become a lifelong habit, it can eventually replace keto and help you still keep the pounds off. You can use keto to get thin fast and then start using IF to keep thin in the future. There is no need to stay on keto forever if you don't like it.

The final and biggest benefit is that IF teaches you not to overeat and overcome cravings. Thus, it prepares your mind for the effort required to stick to the keto eating plan. It also enables you to ignore cravings and control your portions, staying within your macro limits on keto.

Side Effects of Fasting on the Keto Diet

The primary side effect of fasting while on the ketogenic diet involves the keto flu. The keto flu is a collection of nasty symptoms that arise in the first week or so of ketosis, which can be exacerbated by fasting.

Keto flu involves extreme fatigue, irritability, sore muscles, bad breath, feeling cold, and headaches. It can cause women to report smelly vaginal discharge. Usually, this flu goes away in a few days. To tolerate it, you should drink lots of electrolytes and increase your salt intake. Try eating a few days of keto before you try fasting to get over the symptoms naturally.

Of course, fainting, vomiting, hair loss, or extreme pain of any kind, are all worrisome symptoms. Stop your diet and fasting altogether, and get a blood workup at the hospital. Make sure you don't have a severe

44

hormonal or mineral deficiency or any other serious health issues before you start the diet and fasting again.

The point of both keto and fasting is that your blood sugar is meant to go low. But if it goes too low, definitely talk to your doctor. If you are an insulin-dependent diabetic, you want to have your doctor's help to lower your insulin to prevent hypoglycemia.

Many people, particularly women, are prone to plateauing on keto. A fast can help to break that plateau. If your weight loss stalls and you still have not reached your goal weight, consider reevaluating how often you fast and take a longer fast. You might also consider lowering your caloric intake on eating days.

Things to Consider

You want to ensure that you get the appropriate number of calories.

The main issue with combining keto and fasting is that you may not get enough calories, and then you starve. Malnutrition is not the goal here, and it will not lead to healthy weight loss. It can cause hormonal imbalances, organ damage, brain damage, illness, muscle loss, metabolic slowdown, and other issues.

The great thing about fats is that they are filling. Therefore, eating keto meals in your eating windows will help you avoid hunger later on. But many people on keto fail to consider how much fat they are eating, and they tend to skimp on the number of fat calories they require. They spend more time ensuring that they do not eat over twenty grams of carbohydrates, and they do not count fat. Going over or under on fat calories will defeat the diet, so be sure to use a keto calculator free online to find how many macros you need to consume each day. Factors into your diet plan to avoid overeating, hunger, or loss of muscle mass.

Make sure you are getting adequate vitamins and minerals. A daily supplement is a good place to start, but often it doesn't have enough of every element, or it is not absorbed in your body thoroughly. Therefore, you must also get vitamins and minerals from the food you eat. Dairy from calcium, iron from kale or spinach, vitamin D from mushrooms, vitamin C, and beta carotene from carrots and bell peppers, and vitamin E from almonds are all great places to start. In moderation, berries are keto-friendly and contain vitamin C and antioxidants to prevent aging.

Chapter 5. The Most Common Mistakes

Many people who are just starting their fasting cycle, tend to make beginners´ mistakes, which can result in goals not being achieved and many other hosts of things. In this chapter, we will go over the main mistakes most beginners make when they first start fasting. If you are beginning with intermittent fasting, chances are you will make those mistakes. Meaning, for it to not happen, it is best that we talk about it and show you ways to combat it. With that being said, let's talk about the first mistake.

Start Intermittent Fasting Quickly

Many beginners make the mistake of starting intermittent fasting way too fast, and when they begin too quickly, it becomes unsustainable for them to continue with intermittent fasting. If you have started anything immediately, you might have noticed that it became tough for you to follow, which led to you not continuing. The same goes for intermittent fasting, and you need to make sure you take the right steps before you jump into following intermittent fasting. With that being said, let's talk about many ways beginner intermittent fasters tend to start too quickly.

The first mistake they make is by picking a fasting protocol, which is way out of their Realm.

As we talked about before, you need to ease into intermittent fasting, especially if you're a woman. You cannot expect to fast for 24 hours when you have never even fasted in your life, so start small. It is always recommended that women begin with a 12-hour fast, or if that sounds too intense for you can start to by meal skipping. You have to make sure that, whatever you follow is done gradually, so you don't quit. Another way people tend to start intermittent fasting too quickly is by not Consulting the doctor. Believe it or not, their chances that you might not be healthy enough to follow intermittent fasting.

That is why it is advised that you consult a doctor before starting fasting; for example, if you have diabetes, you are not advised to begin intermittent fasting. There are many health complications which not allow you to follow intermittent fasting, that is why we always recommend you ask a doctor before you start intermittent fasting, or it can be very devastating.

Beginners also tend to extend the fasting window very quickly; if you haven't fasted for more than four weeks comfortably, then it is not recommended to extend the fasting window. We need to take into consideration that for beginners, going from 12 hours to 16 hours can be a drastic difference. That is why it is always advised that you stick with a fasting protocol for an extended period, ideally for four weeks. If you make the jump of increasing hours too soon, you will notice it becomes tough for you to continue with fasting, and you might give up.

Choose The Wrong Plan for Your Lifestyle

Most people, when they first start intermittent fasting, tend to pick the crazy strategy for their lifestyle. It is important that you choose the right method for your lifestyle and your goals. Intermittent fasting can be very fitting for most lifestyles. However, some plans are just better suited for some. This is what we are going to be talking about in this section of the book, picking the right plan for your lifestyle. To simplify this process, we will make up two people and make up a fake lifestyle.

Once we have managed to do that, we will figure out which fasting protocol works best for them. The first example would be Jamie, and she is the CEO of a company. Her daily routine is, she wakes up at 5 am and heads on out to her office. She works for 10 hours a day, in and out of meetings, and has barely enough time to go to the bathroom. Her job is physically demanding, and it is also very mentally demanding.

Her goal is to lose a little weight, and she also wants more mental clarity since she has been noticing mental fog sometimes. According to Jamie's lifestyle, it is highly recommended that she follows a fasting protocol that requires less than 24 hours of fasting and is supported regularly.

The reason behind her fasting less than 24 hours, is that when you fast for longer than 24 hours, you tend to notice diminishing results in energy; which is not something we want for Jamie since she has to run a company. On the other hand, she wants less mental fog and more focus.

As you know, fasting for 12 to 20 hours has shown to increase mental focus, which would make a protocol 16/8 or the 12 hours fast more feasible for Jamie. She also wanted to lose weight, which can be done following the 16 hours quickly. In the future, if Jamie wants to lose more weight without losing mental focus, then she can do that by following the warrior diet instead merely because it will shorten her eating window putting her in a higher caloric deficit. To summarize, Jamie's goal was to gain more mental clarity and energy while losing some fat. Her lifestyle is very demanding.

Hence, she is required to be on her "A game" every day, which is why the 12-hour fast or the 16-hour fast will work tremendously, as it has shown to help with mental energy and losing weight. If your lifestyle sounds similar to Jamie's, then I would highly recommend you follow the 12 hours fast or the 16 hours fast. For the next case study, we will pick Amanda. She has two kids, and she works part-time. Her main goal is to lose weight as quickly as possible, but healthily, she has gained a lot of weight after her last pregnancy. Her daily lifestyle is very sedentary since her kids are not infants anymore; taking care of them is more comfortable.

She works from home part-time, and her job is straightforward going. She has had experience with fasting before, she has followed the 12 hours fast and the 16 hours fasts both for 4 weeks. But now, she is dangerous, and she wants to lose a ton of weight quickly. Since Amanda has experience with intermittent fasting, she can go right ahead and follow the 2 days a week fasting protocol or the alternate-day fasting protocol; these two will put her in a 20%–25% deficit for the whole week, making her lose weight quickly and in a healthy manner.

To sum up, Amanda, she has a very sedentary lifestyle. Her goal is to lose the pregnancy weight quickly and to do it healthily, she has followed the 12 hours fast and the 16 hours fast before. Based on her goals and ideally lifestyle, she can start with the alternate fasting protocol or the two days a week fasting protocol. If your goals and lifestyle sound very similar to Amanda's, then you should follow the two days a week fasting protocol or the alternate-day fasting protocol. Hopefully, these two examples helped you understand which fasting protocol is best suited for your lifestyle. Just remember that fasting will only help you if you can do it for a sustained period, which is why lifestyle plays a huge role in sustainability for intermittent fasting. Pick your fasting protocols accordingly.

Overeat During the Eating Window or Too Little

People make the mistake of eating a lot or too little when following intermittent fasting, and the truth is it is straightforward to do either. People who are looking to lose weight will eat less during their eating window, thinking that it will help you lose more body fat. Whereas overeating will not make up for all the fasting, you did throughout the day. This is why it is imperative that you do none, so in this section, we will teach you how to make sure you aren't doing either when following an intermittent fasting protocol.

The first way to not mess up on overeating would be to make sure that you are counting your macros. This is one of the best ways to make sure you stay on track with your eating habits during your fasting windows. When you have calculated your macros and following them accordingly, you will have a lot better chance of not under-eating or overeating during your eating window. Another way to make sure that you are not overeating is to eat slowly, and many people tend to get extremely excited when they see food in front of them during their eating window. It is best advised that you don't indulge in them and more than you should.

That is why it is essential that you control your cravings. Now, even though fasting allows you to eat whatever you want when you break your fast, it is still essential to make sure you eat correctly. You see, if you try and eat junk food and try and hit your macros, it would be tough for you not to overeat. Let me explain how that works, as there is something called a high glycemic carb which is most of the junk foods. These high glycemic carbs are responsible for digesting very quickly in your body, which spikes the insulin very fast.

When you absorb and shuttle the foods to quickly as you would with junk food, you will get hungry very fast, which would make you overeat. This is why it is best advised that you eat foods that have a lower glycemic index like most healthy meals tend to have. Another thing these healthy foods will help you with would be the fiber, making you feel fuller through the day. Now that we know how not to overeat, let's talk about how to make sure that you aren't under-eating. The first way to make sure that you aren't under-eating would be by counting macros, and this will help you make sure that you are hitting all your calories for the day. Counting macros will ensure you don't under-eat and you don't overeat, it goes hand in hand.

Now, this is the only way to avoid under-eating, let's talk about some of the signs you might be experiencing if you under-eat when fasting. The first sign you might notice is that you feel very weak when working out, if you follow a workout plan, you will see that your strength has gone down, which is a tail-tail sign that you are under-eating. Another way to tell that you are under-eating is if you know that you feel less energy throughout the day, rather than feeling more heat. One of the many benefits of intermittent fasting is the fact that you can get a lot more power, but it won't work if you are under-eating. So, by now, you can tell that overeating and under-eating aren't optimal for fasting. This is why you need to make sure that you stay on track with your macros when fasting, the other tips we gave you work great as well.

But do whatever works for you to ensure that you aren't under-eating or overeating, and there are millions of ways to go about it. Find an eating routine that helps you feel full, and allows you to eat just the right number of calories to where you are getting closer to your goals, instead of drifting away from them, if your goal is weight loss or muscle gains, you need to make sure your calories are the right amount. Don't make this beginners´ mistake as you will regret it, and now you have the tools to ensure you don't make these mistakes.

Ignore What for When

One mistake that many people following intermittent fasting make is to ignore what for when. For you to be successful with intermittent fasting, you need to make sure you don't overlook what for when. What do I mean by what for when is simple, ignoring what to do and what not to do when intermittent fasting. We will talk about things to avoid and the things not to avoid when intermittent fasting. More specifically, we will teach you how to listen to your body.

You are ignoring what for when is merely a metaphor, nonetheless an important one. First of all, when intermittent fasting doesn't jump too quickly from fasts to fasts. Most beginners make the mistake of not riding out the protocol for a substantial amount of time before they jump to conclusions. Make sure that you have done at least four weeks of following this protocol, as it will show you how your body reacts to this fasting method. The next thing to make sure of would be to understand how your body reacts to certain types of fasting, as it is essential that you know so.

Before you jump the guns of upping the fasting difficultly, make sure you know how your body works. You need to remember that your body is more important than your goals, so whatever you do, you need to be aware of what your body is telling you. Don't do anything which makes you feel like you are harming your body, and as always, consult with your physician before you start a fast.

Not Drinking Enough Water

Drinking water is crucial when your intermittent fasting, there are a lot of benefits to drinking water. It also helps you care about your appetite. We will talk about the reasons why you should be drinking more water when intermittent fasting, and also show you why you might not be drinking enough water and techniques to allow you to drink more water when fasting. Many people know that water is very beneficial to humans, water helps to detox your body clean out your system, and also helps you curb appetite. It is crucial that you're drinking more water when fasting. Believe it or not, most of the time you're drinking a lot less water than you are required to be drinking. One of the best rules of thumb to follow when you are drinking water is to drink 1 oz. per pound of body weight. So, if you weigh 150 lbs., you should be drinking 150 oz. of water, especially when you're intermittent fasting; as water will help you forget about food.

Many people know that when you're fasting, especially in the beginning, you tend to crave a lot of food. What water will do is help you curb that appetite, so you don't break you're fast prematurely, another thing water will do detoxify your body. When you're fasting, you're already detoxing a lot of things, if you add more water to it, it will help you detox your body even further, making it a lot healthier environment for you. Water will also increase your brain power and productivity, as you know, intermittent fasting has been shown to improve mental focus, so once you add more water to your daily routine, you will notice more focused throughout the day.

Another thing water helps you with is that it helps you lose body weight. If you started intermittent fasting in the hopes of losing weight, then you need to drink more water. What water does, is to increase your metabolism, which equals more calories burnt throughout the day. Water will also help you clean out your complexion, so if that's what you're looking for, the water will help you with that. Intermittent fasting has been shown to improve your digestive system, but once you add a sufficient amount of water to it will boost it further. Many people know that regularity is the essential thing when it comes to a healthy body, why do I help you with consistency, which will equal a better digestive system and overall well-being. Water will also help you boost your immune system, as it enables you to clean out your toxins.

When incorporated with intermittent fasting, drink more water to boost your immune system. When fasting, you might notice headaches, especially in the beginning, if you drink a sufficient amount of water throughout the day, you will not see problems. Headaches are one of the biggest concerns when fasting, many people notice problems, and to avoid that you should start drinking more water. Another matter that you might see when fasting is cramped, more specifically, muscle cramps. One of the ways to prevent it is to drink more water. Now I can keep going on with the benefits of drinking more water, but you get the idea to drink more water to avoid side effects from fasting that you might see.

One of the ways to ensure that you drink more water is to buy a water bottle with markings on it. First, figure out how much water you need throughout the day and make sure you achieve your goal of drinking a set amount of water. Another way to ensure that you drink more water is to set alarms. What many people do, set alerts on this Smartphone, and when the alarm goes off the drink a glass of water. You can do the same thing to ensure they drink enough water throughout the day, calculate the number of glasses you need to achieve your water intake goal, and then set your timer.

Chapter 6. Simple Examples of Fish-Based Meals

1. Lemon Baked Salmon

Preparation Time: 5 minutes

Cooking time: 20 minutes

Servings: 2

Ingredients:

- 12 oz. salmon filets
- 2 lemons, sliced thinly
- 2 tbsps. Olive oil
- Salt and black pepper, to taste
- 3 sprigs thyme

Directions:

1. Preheat the oven to 350°F.
2. Place half the sliced lemons on the bottom of a baking dish.
3. Place the fillets over the lemons and cover with the remaining lemon slices and thyme.

4. Drizzle olive oil over the dish, and cook for 20 minutes.

5. Season with salt and pepper.

Nutrition:

- **Calories:** 571 kcal
- **Fat:** 44 g
- **Fiber:** 2 g
- **Carbs:** 2 g
- **Protein:** 42 g

2. Seafood Casserole

Preparation Time: 30 minutes

Cooking time: 35 minutes

Servings: 6

Ingredients:

Poached Seafood:

- 1 cup dry white wine
- 1 cup water
- 2 small bay leaves, whole
- ½ tsp. old bay seasoning
- 12 oz. shrimp, thawed, peeled, and deveined
- 12 oz. cod, diced

Vegetables:

- 2 stalks celery, diced
- 2 tbsp. butter
- 2 medium leeks, white part only, sliced
- Sea salt, to taste

Sauce:

- ½ tsp. xanthan gum

- 1 cup heavy whipping cream

- 1 tbsp. butter

- ¼ tsp. sea salt

Topping:

- 1 tbsp. butter

- 4 oz. Parmesan cheese, shredded

- 2 tsp. old bay seasoning

- ¼ cup almond flour

- 1 tbsp. fresh parsley, chopped

Directions:

1. Set the oven's temperature at 400°F to preheat.

2. Take a large-sized saucepan and place it over medium-high heat.

3. Add dry white wine, bay leaves, water, and ½ tsp. old bay to the saucepan.

4. Cook the mixture for 3 minutes on a simmer.

5. Add shrimp to the wine mixture and cook until the shrimp changes color.

6. Remove the shrimp from the poaching liquid using a slotted spoon and transfer it to a plate.

7. Add cod to the poaching liquid and cook until the fish turns white.

8. Remove the codfish from the liquid and keep it aside on a plate.

9. Cook the poaching liquid until it is reduced to 1 cup.

10. Take a Dutch oven and place it over medium-high heat.

11. Add 2 tbsp. butter to the Dutch oven and melt it.

12. Stir in leeks and celery, then stir-fry until soft.

13. Season the vegetables with sea salt, then remove from heat.

14. Spread the vegetables in a casserole dish, then toss in the seafood.

15. Add sauce ingredients to the same Dutch oven and cook, stirring until it thickens.

16. Pour the sauce over the seafood in the casserole dish.

17. Prepare the topping by blending almond flour with 1 tbsp. butter, 2 tsp. old bay, and Parmesan cheese.

18. Spread this crumble over the seafood mixture, then bake for 20 minutes in the oven.

19. Serve warm and fresh.

Nutrition:

- **Calories:** 292 kcal
- **Total Fat:** 12.9 g
- **Saturated Fat:** 7.7 g
- **Carbohydrate:** 3.6 g
- **Dietary Fiber:** 0.1 g
- **Sugars:** 0.5 g
- **Protein:** 32.5 g

3. Shrimp Scampi

Preparation Time: 20 minutes

Cooking time: 12 minutes

Servings: 6

Ingredients:

- 1 ¼ lb. shrimp, peeled and deveined
- 4 tbsp. butter
- 3 garlic cloves, roughly chopped
- ¼ cup Chardonnay
- ¼ cup lemon juice
- ¼ tsp. red pepper flakes
- ¼ cup parsley, chopped
- 2 scallions, sliced
- ½ cup Parmesan cheese, shredded
- Salt and black pepper, to taste
- 1 oz. cherry tomatoes, halved

Directions:

1. Peel and devein the shrimp and keep them ready aside.
2. Finely chop the parsley and garlic.
3. Take a large-sized sauté pan and place it over medium heat.

4. Add butter to the pan and heat it to melt.

5. Stir in garlic and sauté until soft.

6. Toss in shrimp and stir-fry until they turn pink.

7. Flip the shrimp and season with red pepper flakes.

8. Add lemon juice and wine, then cook until the liquid is reduced.

9. Remove the shrimp from heat and add parsley.

10. Garnish with Parmesan and serve warm.

Nutrition:

- **Calories:** 210 kcal
- **Total Fat:** 10 g
- **Saturated Fat:** 5.8 g
- **Carbohydrate:** 5.5 g
- **Dietary Fiber:** 0.9 g
- **Sugars:** 2.6 g
- **Protein:** 23.2 g

4. **Easy Blackened Shrimp**

Preparation Time: 10 minutes

Cooking time: 6 minutes

Servings: 2

Ingredients:

- ½ lb. shrimp, peeled and deveined
- 2 tbsp. blackened seasoning
- 1 tsp. olive oil
- Juice of 1 lemon

Directions:

1. Toss all ingredients (except oil) together until shrimp are well coated.
2. In a non-stick skillet, heat the oil to medium-high heat.
3. Add shrimp and cook 2–3 minutes per side.
4. Serve immediately.

Nutrition:

- **Calories:** 152 kcal
- **Fat:** 4 g
- **Fiber:** 1 g
- **Carbs:** 8 g
- **Protein:** 24 g

5. Pan-fried Cod

Preparation Time: 5 minutes

Cooking time: 10 minutes

Servings: 2

Ingredients:

- 12 oz. cod fillet
- 1 tbsp. scallions, chopped
- 1 tbsp. butter
- 1 tbsp. coconut oil
- 1 tsp. garlic, diced
- 1 tsp. cumin seeds
- 1 tsp. coriander seeds
- 1 tsp. salt

Directions:

1. Place butter and coconut oil in the skillet and melt them.
2. Add garlic, cumin, and coriander seeds.
3. Rub the fish fillet with salt and place it in the skillet.
4. Fry the fish for 2 minutes from each side or until it is light brown.
5. Transfer the cooked cod fillet to the plate and cut into 2 servings.

Nutrition:

- **Calories:** 253 kcal
- **Fat:** 14.3 g
- **Fiber:** 0.2 g
- **Carbs:** 1.2 g
- **Protein:** 30.8 g

6. Grilled Shrimp Easy Seasoning

Preparation Time: 5 minutes

Cooking time: 5 minutes

Servings: 4

Ingredients:

Shrimp Seasoning:

- 1 tsp. garlic powder
- 1 tsp. kosher salt
- 1 tsp. Italian seasoning
- ¼ tsp. cayenne pepper

Grilling:

- 2 tbsp. Olive oil
- 1 tbsp. lemon juice
- 1 lb. jumbo shrimp, peeled, deveined
- Ghee for the grill

Directions:

1. Preheat the grill pan to high.
2. In a mixing bowl, stir together the seasoning ingredients.
3. Drizzle in the lemon juice and olive oil and stir.

4. Add the shrimp and toss to coat.

5. Brush the grill pan with ghee.

6. Grill the shrimp until pink, about 2–3 minutes per side.

7. Serve immediately.

Nutrition:

- **Calories:** 101 kcal

- **Fat:** 3 g

- **Fiber:** 1 g

- **Carbs:** 1 g

- **Protein:** 28 g

7. Tuna Casserole

Preparation Time: 5 minutes

Cooking time: 50 minutes

Servings: 4

Ingredients:

- 16 oz. tuna in oil, drained

- 2 tbsp. butter

- ½ tsp. salt

- 1 tsp. black pepper

- 1 tsp. chili powder
- 6 stalks celery
- 1 green bell pepper
- 1 yellow onion
- 4 oz. Parmesan cheese, grated
- 1 cup mayonnaise
- Lard, as needed

Directions:

1. Heat the oven to 400°F. Very finely chop the onion, bell pepper, and celery. Then fry them with the butter for 5 minutes.
2. Add and stir in the chili powder, parmesan cheese, tuna, and mayonnaise. Use some lard to grease an 8x8-inch or 9x9-inch baking pan.
3. Add the tuna mixture into the fried vegetables and spoon the mix into the baking pan.
4. Bake it for 20 minutes.

Nutrition:

- **Calories:** 953 kcal
- **Carbs:** 5 g
- **Fat:** 83 g
- **Protein:** 43 g

8. Mussels with White Wine and Leeks

Preparation Time: 30 minutes

Cooking time: 15 minutes

Servings: 2–4

Ingredients:

- 2 lb. mussels
- 8 cups cold water
- 2 tbsp. sea salt
- 1 small leek
- 1 tbsp. extra-virgin olive oil
- 1 tbsp. butter, unsalted
- 2 garlic cloves, minced
- 4 thyme sprigs
- 1 cup dry white wine
- 1 tbsp. Bone Broth (optional)
- 1 tbsp. fresh parsley, chopped

Directions:

1. Place the mussels in a clean sink full of water. Scrub them with a brush to remove their beards. Rinse and soak again if still gritty. Drain.
2. In a large pot or bowl, combine the mussels, cold water, and salt. Let soak for 10 minutes. Discard any open mussels. Rinse the remaining mussels.
3. Cut the leek lengthwise, remove the greens, and clean well. Chop the white parts medium-fine. Set aside.

4. Prepare a large pot, then heat the oil over medium-low heat, and melt the butter. Add the chopped leek to the pot and cook for 4 to 6 minutes, until softened.

5. Add the garlic and reduce the heat to low. Remove the thyme leaves from the stems and add them to the pot along with the white wine and bone broth (if using). Increase the heat to medium-high.

6. Add the mussels and cover the pot. Steam for 5–7 minutes; if the mussels are open, they're ready. Discard any mussels that don't open. Stir in the fresh parsley. Spoon the mussels and broth into shallow bowls and serve.

Nutrition:

- **Calories:** 632 kcal
- **Total Fat:** 23 g
- **Total Carbohydrates:** 28 g
- **Fiber:** 1 g
- **Sugar:** 3 g
- **Protein:** 55 g
- **Sodium:** 1315 mg

Chapter 7 . Simple Examples of Meat Dishes

9. Pan-Fried Pork Tenderloin

Preparation Time: 5 minutes

Cooking time: 25 minutes

Servings: 2

Ingredients:

- 1 lb. (454 g) pork tenderloin
- Salt and pepper to taste
- 1 tbsp. coconut oil to cook in

Directions:

1. Chop the 1 lb. Pork tenderloin in half.
2. Put the 1 tbsp. coconut oil into a frying pan on medium heat.
3. Bring the 2 pork tenderloin pieces into the pan.
4. Leave the pork to cook. Sprinkle salt and pepper to taste. When that side is cooked, use tongs to turn and to cook the other side.

Continue turning and cooking until the pork looks cooked on all sides.

5. Cook all sides of the pork until the meat thermometer shows an internal temperature of just below 145°F (63°C). The pork will keep on cooking a bit after you pull it out from the pan.

6. Let the pork sit for 1–2 minutes and then slice into 1-inch-thick slices with a sharp knife.

Nutrition:

- **Calories:** 330 kcal
- **Fat:** 15 g
- **Net Carbohydrates:** 0 g
- **Protein:** 47 g

10. Happy Burrito Bowl Pork

Preparation Time: 10 minutes

Cooking time: 5 minutes

Servings: 4

Ingredients:

- 1-½ tbsp. pork lard
- 1 onion, sliced
- 2 bell peppers, sliced
- 1 garlic clove, chopped
- Salt and pepper to taste
- 1 lb. pork, pulled
- ½ cup chicken pork
- ½ cup chicken broth
- 6 cups lettuce, chopped
- 6 cups cabbage, chopped
- ¼ cup guacamole

Directions:

1. Set your Ninja Foodi to Sauté mode and add lard, let it melt, and add onion and bell pepper

2. Cook for 2 minutes, stirring for 2 minutes. Add garlic, salt, and pepper

3. Stir well. Add pulled pork and chicken pork

4. Lock lid and cook on high pressure for 1 minute. Quick-release pressure

5. Arrange lettuce and green cabbage in serving bowls, and add pulled pork on top

6. Top with guacamole and serve. Enjoy!

Nutrition:

- **Calories:** 417 kcal
- **Fat:** 95 g
- **Carbohydrates:** 6 g
- **Protein:** 75 g

11.Sauerkraut Pork

Preparation Time: 10 minutes

Cooking time: 35 minutes

Servings: 4

Ingredients:

- 3 lb. pork shoulder
- Salt and pepper to taste
- 3 tbsp. butter
- 2 onions, chopped
- 3 cloves garlic, sliced
- 6 cups sauerkraut, divided
- 1-lb. hot dog, sliced and cooked
- ½ lb. kielbasa, sliced and cooked

Directions:

1. Season pork roast with salt and pepper.
2. Set your Ninja Foodi to Sauté mode and add butter, let the butter melt.
3. Add pork roast and brown. Pour 2 cups water, onion, and garlic.
4. Season with salt and pepper and close the lid. Cook on high pressure for 35 minutes.

5. Release pressure naturally over 10 minutes.

6. Shred pork and stir in sauerkraut, hotdog, and kielbasa. Serve and enjoy!

Nutrition:

- **Calories:** 792 kcal
- **Fat:** 83 g
- **Carbohydrates:** 14g
- **Protein:** 68 g

12.Roasted Pork Loin with Grainy Mustard Sauce

Preparation Time: 10 minutes

Cooking time: 70 minutes

Servings: 8

Ingredients:

- 1 (2-lb.) pork loin roast, boneless
- Sea salt
- Black pepper, freshly ground
- 3 tbsp. olive oil
- 1-½ cups heavy (whipping) cream
- 3 tbsp. grainy mustard, such as Pommery

Directions:

1. Set the oven to 375°F.
2. Season the pork roast all over with pepper and sea salt.
3. Bring a large skillet at medium-high heat and add the olive oil.
4. Brown the roast on all sides in the skillet, about 6 minutes in total, and place the roast in a baking dish.

5. Roast until a meat thermometer inserted in the thickest part of the roast reads 155°F, about 1 hour.

6. When approximately 15 minutes of roasting time are left, put a small saucepan at medium heat, then add the heavy cream and mustard.

7. Mix the sauce until it simmers, then lower the heat. Simmer the sauce until it is very rich and thick, about 5 minutes. Take off the pan from the heat and set it aside.

8. Allow the pork to rest for around 10 minutes before slicing and serve with the sauce.

Nutrition:

- **Calories:** 368 kcal
- **Fat:** 29 g
- **Protein:** 25 g
- **Carbs:** 2 g
- **Fiber:** 0 g
- **Net Carbs:** 2 g

13.Lamb Chops with Kalamata Tapenade

Preparation Time: 15 minutes

Cooking time: 25 minutes

Servings: 4

Ingredients:

For the tapenade:

- 1 cup Kalamata olives, pitted
- 2 tbsp. fresh parsley, chopped
- 2 tbsp. extra-virgin olive oil
- 2 tsp. garlic, minced
- 2 tsp. lemon juice, freshly squeezed

For the Lamb Chops:

- 2 (1-lb.) racks French-cut lamb chops (8 bones each)
- Sea salt
- Black pepper, freshly ground
- 1-tbsp. olive oil

Directions:

To make the Tapenade:

1. Place the olives, parsley, olive oil, garlic, and lemon juice in a food processor, and process until the mixture is puréed, but still slightly chunky.
2. Transfer the tapenade to a container and store sealed in the refrigerator until needed.

To make the Lamb Chops:

1. Preheat the oven to 450°F.
2. Season the lamb racks with salt and pepper.
3. Put a large ovenproof skillet over medium-high heat and add the olive oil.
4. Pan sear the lamb racks on all sides until browned, about 5 minutes in total.
5. Arrange the racks upright in the skillet, with the bones interlaced, and roast them in the oven until they reach your desired doneness, about 20 minutes for medium-rare or until the internal temperature reaches 125°F.
6. Allow the lamb to rest for around 10 minutes, and then cut the lamb racks into chops. Arrange 4 chops per person on the plate and top with the Kalamata tapenade.

Nutrition:

- **Calories:** 348 kcal
- **Fat:** 28 g
- **Protein:** 21 g
- **Carbs:** 2 g
- **Fiber:** 1 g
- **Net Carbs:** 1 g

14.Bacon Wrapped-Beef Tenderloin

Preparation Time: 10 minutes

Cooking time: 15 minutes

Servings: 4

Ingredients:

- 4 (4-oz.) beef tenderloin steaks
- Sea salt
- Black pepper, freshly ground
- 8 bacon slices
- 1 tbsp. extra-virgin olive oil

Directions:

1. Preheat the oven to 450°F.
2. Season the steaks with salt and pepper.
3. Wrap each steak snugly around the edges with 2 slices of bacon and secure the bacon with toothpicks.
4. Bring a large skillet at medium-high heat and add the olive oil.
5. Pan sear the steaks for 4 minutes per side and transfer them to a baking sheet.
6. Roast the steaks until they reach your desired doneness, about 6 minutes for medium.

7. Remove the steaks from the oven and let them rest for 10 minutes.

8. Remove the toothpicks and serve.

Nutrition:

- **Calories:** 565 kcal
- **Fat:** 49 g
- **Protein:** 28 g
- **Carbs:** 0 g
- **Fiber:** 0 g
- **Net Carbs:** 0 g

15. Butter Chicken

Preparation Time: 5 minutes

Cooking time: 30 minutes

Servings: 4

Ingredients:

- ¼ cup butter
- 2 cups mushrooms, sliced
- 4 large chicken thighs
- ½ tsp. onion powder
- ½ tsp. garlic powder
- 1 tsp. kosher salt
- ¼ tsp. black pepper
- ½ cup water
- 1 tsp. Dijon mustard
- 1 tbsp. fresh tarragon, chopped

Directions:

1. Season the chicken thighs with onion powder, garlic powder, salt, and pepper.
2. In a sauté pan, melt 1 tbsp. butter.

3. Sear the chicken thighs for about 3 to 4 minutes per side, or until both sides are golden brown. Remove the thighs from the pan.

4. Add the remaining 3 tbsp. butter to the pan and melt.

5. Add the mushrooms and cook for 4 to 5 minutes or until golden brown. Stirring as little as possible.

6. Add the Dijon mustard and water to the pan. Stir to deglaze.

7. Place the chicken thighs back in the pan with the skin side up.

8. Cover and simmer for 15 minutes.

9. Stir in the fresh herbs. Let sit for 5 minutes and serve.

Nutrition:

- **Calories:** 414 kcal
- **Fat:** 9 g
- **Fiber:** 2 g
- **Carbs:** 2 g
- **Protein:** 27 g

16.Slow-Cooked Salsa Chicken

Preparation Time: 5 minutes

Cooking time: 2 hours

Servings: 6

Ingredients:

- 3 lb. chicken breasts, boneless, skinless
- 2 cups mild salsa
- 1 cup Mexican Blend cheese, shredded

Direction:

1. Place the chicken in your slow cooker and add the mild salsa.
2. Cover with a lid. Cook on "High" for 1 hour and 30 minutes to 2 hours.
3. Preheat your oven to 425°F.
4. Transfer the chicken to a greased baking dish and sprinkle with the Mexican blend cheese.
5. Place inside your oven and bake for 15 minutes or until golden brown.
6. Serve and enjoy!

Nutrition:

- **Calories:** 351 kcal
- **Fat:** 9 g
- **Fiber:** 1 g
- **Carbs:** 8 g
- **Protein:** 54 g

17.Chicken with Mustard Sauce and Bacon

Preparation Time: 10 minutes

Cooking time: 30 minutes

Servings: 3

Ingredients:

- 2 lb. chicken breast, boneless and skinless
- ⅓ cup Dijon mustard
- ¼ tsp. fine sea salt
- ¼ tsp. paprika, smoked or regular paprika
- 8 medium bacon slices, finely chopped
- 1 small white or red onion, finely chopped
- 1 tbsp. extra-virgin olive oil
- 1 ½ cups homemade low-sodium chicken broth

Direction:

1. In a small bowl, add the Dijon mustard, smoked paprika, fine sea salt, and freshly cracked black pepper. Stir until well combined.
2. Baste the Dijon mustard mixture all over the chicken breast.
3. In a large skillet over medium-high heat, add the bacon and cook until brown and crispy. Transfer to a plate lined with paper towels.

4. Add 1 tbsp. extra-virgin olive oil to the skillet. Add the chicken and cook for 2 minutes per side. Transfer the chicken to a plate.

5. Pour the chicken broth into the skillet and raise the heat until begins to bubble. Return the cooked bacon and chopped onions to the skillet.

6. Return the chicken to the skillet and reduce the heat. Cover with a lid and allow to simmer for 15 to 20 minutes or until the chicken is thoroughly cooked.

7. Serve and enjoy!

Nutrition:

- **Calories:** 681 kcal
- **Fat:** 9 g
- **Fiber:** 2 g
- **Carbs:** 8 g
- **Protein:** 74 g

18. Beef Satay with Vegetables

Preparation Time: 10 minutes

Cooking time: 50 minutes

Servings: 4

Ingredients:

- Flank steak, cut into ¼-inch strips
- 2 tsp. paste Thai red curry
- ½ tsp. fresh ginger, ground
- ¼ cup milk from coconuts
- 1 tsp. monk fruit sweetener, granulated
- ¼ cup natural butter of peanuts
- 2 tsp. soy sauce low sodium
- 1 tsp. lime juice
- 1 tsp. olive oil extra virgin
- 2 cauliflower heads, grated
- ¼ tsp. salt
- ¼ tsp. powder of black pepper, freshly ground
- 1 cup green beans

Directions:

1. Heat an indoor grill in advance.
2. Get a container used for mixing, and in it mix the milk from coconuts, natural butter from peanuts, sauce of soy, a sweetener from monk fruits, Thai paste, and fresh ginger that has been ground.

3. Divide the above mix into 2 separate containers and in 1, add in the flank steak strips.

4. Let the flank steak marinate in the sauce for half an hour.

5. While waiting for foot, the flank steak to marinate, take a non-stick skillet and add the olive oil extra virgin into it.

6. When the oil is nice and hot, add in the grated cauliflower together with black pepper that is freshly ground and salt to season it. Let this cook for 5 minutes.

7. Take the cooked cauliflower from the pan, and in it, add some more olive oil and fry the green beans for 5 minutes when they will appear to have a bright green color on them and are not too tender.

8. Take the marinated flanks of steak and grill them on an indoor grill you had heated in advance for about 3 minutes.

9. When ready, serve the grilled flanks of steak with the cooked cauliflower and green beans as well.

Nutrition:

- **Calories:** 191 kcal
- **Fat:** 9 g
- **Fiber:** 2 g
- **Carbs:** 8 g
- **Protein:** 20 g

19.Parmesan Chicken with Zucchini

Preparation Time: 10 minutes

Cooking time: 20 minutes

Servings: 6

Ingredients:

- 2 cups chicken, minced
- 4 big zucchinis, halved along their length
- Low-carb tomato basil sauce
- 3 tbsp. olive oil extra virgin
- ¼ cup parmesan cheese, grated
- Small yellow onion, diced
- ¼ cup mozzarella cheese, grated
- 2 garlic cloves, minced
- 1 tsp. basil, dried
- ¼ tsp. salt
- ¼ tsp. black pepper powder, freshly ground

Directions:

1. Preheat your oven to 400°F.
2. Get a large pan used for baking and coat its bottom with the low-carb tomato basil sauce.

3. Get a melon scooper, and with care, scoop out the flesh of the zucchini. Take this flesh and blend it gently in a blender.

4. Take a large pan used for frying and add olive oil extra virgin in it. Heat the oil over medium heat and when it is hot, add in the diced yellow onion. Let the onion fry for 3 minutes, then add in the minced garlic and cook this for 1 minute until the garlic is fragrant.

5. Pour in the minced chicken and the blended flesh of zucchini. Season this with the black pepper powder freshly ground and salt. Cover and let this cook for 5 minutes until the chicken is well cooked. Pour out the excess fluid that may remain after the chicken is cooked.

6. Take a little of the sauce and pour it into the cooked chicken, stirring so that it covers all the chicken. Let this mixture simmer over medium heat for around 8 minutes.

7. Take the zucchini that has been halved and scooped and place them on a plate. Scoop the minced chicken mixture and place it in the middle of the halved zucchini. Take the stuffed zucchini pieces and place them on the dish for baking you prepared earlier.

8. Cover the dish with foil and place it in the oven you had heated in advance. Let them bake in the oven for 25 minutes when the zucchini softens.

9. When the zucchini is soft, take the dish for baking from the oven and unwrap the foil. Sprinkle the grated parmesan and

mozzarella cheese at the top. Put back the dish for baking in the oven and let it bake until all the cheese melts well.

10. Take it from the oven and serve.

Nutrition:

- **Calories:** 267 kcal
- **Fat:** 34 g
- **Fiber:** 2 g
- **Carbs:** 8 g
- **Protein:** 46 g

20.Pork Lettuce Wraps

Preparation Time: 15 minutes

Cooking time: 20 minutes

Servings: 2

Ingredients:

- 9 oz. pork, ground
- 6 black olives, pitted and sliced
- 2 oz. bell pepper
- 5 tbsp. spring onions, chopped
- 4 leaves romaine lettuce
- 1 ½ tbsp. sour cream
- ½ avocado, peeled and pitted, cubed
- 1 tbsp. olive oil
- ¼ tsp. black pepper
- ½ tsp. chili flakes
- ½ tsp. paprika
- 2 tbsp. parsley for garnish
- Salt to taste

Directions:

1. Take a large pan, add the olive oil, and put it over medium heat. Cut the peppers into thin slices. Add peppers to the pan and cook it for 2–3 minutes or until you see it softened. Remove bell peppers to a plate and set them aside.

2. Put the ground pork into the pan and fry until browned all over.

3. Sprinkle pork with all the seasonings, salt, and spring onions. Stir everything well and continue cooking until the pork is done.

4. Take lettuce leaves and divide the entire mixture between them. Put bell peppers on top.

5. Pour the sour cream over the pork and toss in sliced olives, cubed avocado, and chopped parsley. Your meal is ready to serve.

Nutrition:

- **Calories:** 566 kcal
- **Total Carbs:** 9 g
- **Fiber:** 5 g
- **Net Carbs:** 4 g
- **Fat:** 44 g
- **Protein:** 35 g

21.Cabbage and Bacon Bake

Preparation Time: 10 minutes

Cooking time: 25 minutes

Servings: 4

Ingredients:

- 1 oz. bacon
- 2 tbsp. heavy cream
- 1 tbsp. cream cheese
- 3 oz. cheddar cheese, shredded
- 1 tbsp. olive oil
- ½ cup water
- 18 oz. cabbage, chopped in half-inch strips
- ½ garlic clove
- 1 tbsp. butter
- ½ tsp. black pepper, ground
- Salt to taste

Directions:

1. Take a pan, pour the water, and boil it. Toss in half-inch strips of cabbage and cook for 3–4 minutes or until the cabbage gets softer. Drain it and put it aside.

2. Prepare the oven and preheat it to 400°F.

3. Meanwhile, take a skillet and put olive oil over medium-high heat. Take bacon and fry it until it's crispy. Put it on a plate aside.

4. Take a small pan, melt the butter over low heat and toss in some chopped garlic.

5. Add heavy cream, half of the cheddar cheese, water, and cream cheese. Cook everything to a simmer for 1–2 minutes or until you see sauce thickened and became creamy.

6. Spread cabbage pieces all over a baking dish and add the bacon. Season everything with some pepper and salt.

7. Pour the sauce over bacon and cabbage. Add the remaining cheddar cheese.

8. Place everything in the preheated oven, then bake it for around 18 minutes or until you see the mixture became golden brown.

Nutrition:

- **Calories:** 243 kcal
- **Total Carbs:** 9 g
- **Fiber:** 3 g
- **Net Carbs:** 6 g
- **Fat:** 20 g
- **Protein:** 9 g

22.Sunday Ground Pork Bake

Preparation Time: 9 minutes

Cooking time: 21 minutes

Servings: 4

Ingredients:

- 1 tbsp. butter
- 2 lbs. pork, ground
- 1 bell pepper, deseeded and chopped
- 1 serrano pepper, deseeded and chopped
- 1 leek, chopped
- 2 garlic cloves, minced
- ½ cup chicken broth
- 2 eggs, beaten
- 1 tsp. paprika
- Sea salt, to taste
- Black pepper, ground, to taste
- ½ cup cream cheese
- 1 cup heavy whipped cream

Directions:

1. Melt the butter in a frying pan at moderate heat. Now, cook the ground pork until no longer pink.
2. Add in the peppers, leek, and garlic and continue to cook approximately 7 minutes or until tender and aromatic.
3. Pour the chicken broth and continue to cook for a further 6 minutes. Scoop the mixture into a lightly greased baking pan.
4. In a mixing bowl, whisk the egg, paprika, salt, black pepper, cream cheese, and heavy whipped cream. Pour the mixture into the prepared baking pan.
5. Bake in the preheated oven at 330°F for about 8 minutes until golden brown on the top. Bon appétit!

Nutrition:

- **Calories:** 620 kcal
- **Fat:** 50 g
- **Carbs:** 5.7 g
- **Protein:** 33.9 g
- **Fiber:** 0.7 g

Chapter 8 . Simple Examples of Vegan Dishes

23.Steamed Artichoke

Preparation Time: 5 minutes

Cooking time: 20 minutes

Servings: 4

Ingredients:

- 2 medium artichokes
- 1 lemon
- 2 tbsp. mayonnaise
- 1 tsp. Dijon mustard
- 1 pinch paprika

Directions:

1. Wash properly and remove the harmed outside leaves. On the off threat that the artichokes are barbed, removed the top side and, making use of kitchen shears, trim the spines off the encompassing leaves.

2. Wipe any reduced edges with a lemon ½, this will protect them from oxidizing.

3. In case your artichoke accompanied a stem absolutely cut it off to make a degree base for the artichoke.

4. Strip and reduce the stem and bubble it in the steaming fluid under the artichoke.

5. Add 1 cup of water to the cooker base and lower the steamer bin inside.

6. When time is up, open the cooker with the Natural discharge method, get the cooker off the burner and let it cool.

7. Blend mayonnaise in with mustard and spot in the little plunging compartment, sprinkle with paprika. Serve warm.

Nutrition:

- **Calories:** 77.5 kcal
- **Fat:** 5 g
- **Carbs:** 3.5 g
- **Protein:** 2 g

24.Cauliflower Cups

Preparation Time: 5 minutes

Cooking time: 30 minutes

Servings: 6

Ingredients:

- 1 ½ cups cauliflower rice
- ¼ cup onion, diced
- ½ cup pepper jack cheese, shredded
- ½ tsp. oregano, dried
- ½ tsp. basil, dried
- ½ tsp. salt
- 1 large egg, lightly beaten

Directions:

1. Preheat the oven to 350°F.
2. Put and mix all ingredients in a bowl.
3. Scoop mixture into the wells of a mini muffin tin and pack lightly.
4. Bake for 30 minutes.
5. Cool and serve.

Nutrition:

- **Calories:** 60 kcal
- **Fat:** 3.9 g
- **Carbs:** 1.8 g
- **Protein:** 4.3 g

25. Parmesan Roasted Cabbage

Preparation Time: 5 minutes

Cooking time: 20 minutes

Servings: 4

Ingredients:

- 1 large head green cabbage
- 4 tbsp. butter, melted
- 1 tsp. garlic powder
- Salt and black pepper to taste
- 1 cup Parmesan cheese, grated
- Parmesan cheese, grated, for topping
- 1 tbsp. parsley, chopped, to garnish

Directions:

1. Set the oven to 400°F, line the baking sheet using foil, and grease with cooking spray.
2. Stand the cabbage and run a knife from the top to bottom to cut the cabbage into wedges. Remove stems and wilted leaves. Mix the butter, garlic, salt, and black pepper until evenly combined.
3. Brush the mixture on every side of the cabbage wedges and sprinkle with Parmesan cheese.

4. Put on the baking sheet, then bake for at least 20 minutes to soften the cabbage and melt the cheese. Remove the cabbages when golden brown, plate, and sprinkle with extra cheese and parsley. Serve warm with pan-glazed tofu.

Nutrition:

- **Calories:** 268 kcal
- **Fat:** 19.3 g
- **Net Carbs:** 4 g
- **Protein:** 17.5 g

26. Briam with Tomato Sauce

Preparation Time: 10 minutes

Cooking time: 70 minutes

Servings: 4

Ingredients:

- 3 tbsp. olive oil
- 1 large eggplant, halved and sliced
- 1 large onion, thinly sliced
- 3 cloves garlic, sliced
- 5 tomatoes, diced
- 3 rutabagas, diced
- 1 cup sugar-free tomato sauce
- 4 zucchinis, sliced
- ¼ cup water
- Salt and black pepper to taste
- 1 tbsp. oregano, dried
- 2 tbsp. parsley, chopped

Directions:

1. Preheat the oven to 400°F. Warm the olive oil in a skillet at medium heat and cook the eggplant for 6 minutes until on the

edges. After, remove to a medium bowl. Sauté the onion and garlic in the oil for 3 minutes, and add them to the eggplants. Turn the heat off.

2. In the eggplant bowl, mix in the tomatoes, rutabagas, tomato sauce, and zucchinis. Add the water and stir in the salt, black pepper, oregano, and parsley. Pour the mixture into the casserole dish. Place the dish in the oven and bake for 45 to 60 minutes. Serve the briam warm on a bed of cauli rice.

Nutrition:

- **Calories:** 365 kcal
- **Fat:** 12 g
- **Net Carbs:** 12.5 g
- **Protein:** 11.3 g

27. Grated Cauliflower with Seasoned Mayo

Preparation Time: 10 minutes

Cooking time: 15 minutes

Servings: 2

Ingredients:

- 1 lb. cauliflower, grated
- 3 oz. butter
- 4 eggs
- 3 oz. Padron peppers or poblano peppers
- ½ cup mayonnaise
- 1 tsp. olive oil
- Salt and pepper
- 1 tsp. garlic powder (optional)

Directions:

1. In a bowl, place the mayonnaise and garlic, then whisk and set aside.
2. Rinse, trim, then grate the cauliflower using a food processor or grater.

3. Melt a generous amount of butter and fry grated cauliflower for about 5 minutes. Season salt and pepper to taste.

4. Fry poblanos with oil until lightly crispy. Then fry eggs as you want and sprinkle salt and pepper over them.

5. Serve with poblanos and cauliflower. Drizzle some mayo mixture on top.

Nutrition:

- **Calories:** 898 kcal
- **Fat:** 87 g
- **Carbohydrates:** 9 g
- **Protein:** 17g

28.Oven Roasted Cabbage Wedges

Preparation Time: 15 minutes

Cooking time: 45 minutes

Servings: 4

Ingredients:

- Head green cabbage
- ¼ cup olive oil
- 1 ½ tsp. garlic salt
- 1 tsp. onion powder
- 1 tsp. fennel seeds
- ¼ tsp. black pepper

Directions:

1. Preheat the stove to 400°F. Prepare a baking tray with line paper.
2. Cut the cabbage in 1-inch cuts through and through.
3. Cut lines in a solitary layer on a preparing sheet. Brush each wedge with a liberal covering of olive oil.
4. In a little bowl, consolidate garlic salt, onion powder, fennel seeds, and dark pepper. Sprinkle flavoring over each wedge.
5. Prepare for 45 minutes on the center rack–flipping part of the way through.

Nutrition:

- **Calories:** 120 kcal
- **Fat:** 9 g
- **Carbs:** 2.8 g
- **Protein:** 2 g

29.Paprika Roasted Radishes with Onions

Preparation Time: 20 minutes

Cooking time: 20 minutes

Servings: 4

Ingredients:

- 2 large bunches radishes
- 1 small onion
- 2 tbsp. butter and 2 tbsp. olive oil
- 1 Tsp. fennel seeds
- ½ tsp. paprika, smoked
- Sea salt and black pepper to taste

Directions:

1. Preheat the oven to 350°F. Prepare a baking tray with line paper.
2. In a blending bowl, consolidate radishes and onion. To the bowl, include spread, olive oil, fennel seeds, paprika, ocean salt, and dark pepper. Remove until radishes and onions are uniformly covered.
3. Pour radishes and onions in a solitary layer onto the material paper. Pour any additional spread and flavoring over the top.
4. Prepare for 20 minutes.

Nutrition:

- **Calories:** 289 kcal
- **Fat:** 21.8 g
- **Carbs:** 3.2 g
- **Protein:** 12.3 g

30.Cheesy Roasted Vegetable Spaghetti

Preparation Time: 10 minutes

Cooking time: 35 minutes

Servings: 4

Ingredients:

- 2 (8 oz.) packs shirataki spaghetti
- 1 cup mixed bell peppers, chopped
- ½ cup Parmesan cheese, grated, for topping
- 1 lb. asparagus, chopped
- 1 cup broccoli florets
- 1 cup green beans, chopped
- 3 tbsp. olive oil
- 1 small onion, chopped
- 2 garlic cloves, minced
- 1 cup tomatoes, diced
- ½ cup basil, chopped

Directions:

1. Boil 2 cups of water in a pot. Strain the shirataki pasta and rinse well under hot running water. Allow draining and pour the shirataki pasta into the boiling water.

2. Cook for 3 minutes and strain again. Place a dry skillet and stir-fry the shirataki pasta until visibly dry, 1–2 minutes; set aside.

3. Preheat the oven to 425°F. In a bowl, add asparagus, broccoli, bell peppers, and green beans and toss with half of the olive oil. Bring the vegetables on a baking sheet and roast for 20 minutes.

4. Heat the remaining olive oil in a skillet and sauté onion and garlic for 3 minutes. Stir in tomatoes and cook for 8 minutes.

5. Mix in shirataki and vegetables.

6. Top with Parmesan cheese and serve.

Nutrition:

- **Calories:** 272 kcal
- **Net Carbs:** 7 g
- **Fat:** 12 g
- **Protein:** 12 g

31.Garlic 'n Sour Cream Zucchini Bake

Preparation Time: 10 minutes

Cooking time: 35 minutes

Servings: 3

Ingredients:

- 1 ½ cups zucchini slices
- 5 tbsp. olive oil
- 1 tbsp. garlic, minced
- ¼ cup Parmesan cheese, grated
- 1 (8 oz.) package cream cheese, softened
- Salt and pepper to taste

Directions:

1. Lightly grease a baking sheet using cooking spray.
2. Place zucchini in a bowl and put in olive oil and garlic.
3. Place zucchini slices in a single layer in a dish.
4. Bake for 35 minutes at 390°F until crispy.
5. In a bowl, whisk well, remaining ingredients.
6. Serve with zucchini.

Nutrition:

- **Calories:** 385 kcal
- **Fat:** 32.4 g
- **Carbs:** 9.5 g
- **Protein:** 11.9 g

32. Paprika 'n Cajun Seasoned Onion Rings

Preparation Time: 15 minutes

Cooking time: 25 minutes

Servings: 6

Ingredients:

- 1 large white onion
- 2 large eggs, beaten
- ½ tsp. Cajun seasoning
- ¾ cup almond flour
- 1 ½ tsp. paprika
- ½ cups coconut oil for frying
- ¼ cup water
- Salt and pepper to taste

Directions:

1. Preheat a pot with oil for 8 minutes.
2. Peel the onion, cut off the top, and slice it into circles.
3. In a mixing bowl, combine the water and the eggs. Season with pepper and salt.
4. Soak the onion in the egg mixture.

5. In another bowl, combine the almond flour, paprika powder, Cajun seasoning, salt, and pepper.

6. Dredge the onion in the almond flour mixture.

7. Place in the pot and cook in batches until golden brown, around 8 minutes per batch.

Nutrition:

- **Calories:** 262 kcal
- **Fat:** 24.1 g
- **Carbs:** 3.9 g
- **Protein:** 2.8 g

33. Grilled Parmesan Eggplant

Preparation Time: 5 minutes

Cooking time: 15 minutes

Servings: 4

Ingredients:

- 1 medium-sized eggplant
- 1 log (1 lb.) fresh mozzarella cheese, cut into 16
- 1 small tomato, cut into 8 slices
- ½ cup Parmesan cheese, shredded
- Fresh basil or parsley, chopped
- ½ tsp. salt
- 1 tbsp. olive oil
- ½ tsp. pepper

Directions:

1. Trim the ends of the eggplant; cut eggplant crosswise into 8 slices. Dust with salt; let stand 5 minutes.
2. Pat the eggplant dry with paper towels; brush each side with oil and sprinkle with pepper. Grill, covered, over medium heat 4–6 minutes on each side or until tender. Remove from grill.

3. Top the eggplant with mozzarella cheese, tomato, and Parmesan cheese. Grill, covered, 1–2 minutes longer or until cheese begins to melt. Top with basil.

Nutrition:

- **Calories:** 449 kcal
- **Fat:** 31 g
- **Carbs:** 10 g
- **Protein:** 26 g

Chapter 9 FAQ

Fasting can be difficult at times, and we know it! There are certain concerns that every beginner gets after opting for intermittent fasting. The following frequently asked questions can help resolve basic queries about fasting and its effects on health.

Question # 1:   Can I Take Bone Broth?

First of all: what is bone broth, and why would anyone be interested in taking it?

In short, bone broth is the drink obtained by boiling the bones and connective tissue of different types of animals.

It is rich in vitamins, minerals, collagen, and other nutrients.

And it is precise because the bone broth is rich in nutrients that it becomes interesting for longer fasts.

Because it has the ability to replace nutrients (vitamins and minerals) lost during the fasting window.

After all, you are frequently eliminating water and minerals during this period through urine and perspiration.

Question # 2:   What Breaks Fasting?

There is no single answer to this case—but calmly, let's explain it properly.

And by the end, you will understand the truth of why some people say that a certain food or drink "breaks" fasting, and why others say it does not.

In fact, the answer to that question is to distinguish between two types of fasting: insulin fasting and calorie fasting.

Insulin fasting:

Insulin Fasting is a type of fasting where you will focus primarily on not raising your insulin.

That is, you will not be able to eat foods that raise insulin, being a little more permissive with foods that do not raise insulin.

And what are these foods that do not raise insulin?

Well, the only macronutrient that doesn't have much effect on insulin is fat.

Because both proteins and carbohydrates cause a certain increase in the levels of this hormone.

Question # 3:   What Can I Eat or Drink during Fasting?

As we said earlier, to reap the full benefits that intermittent fasting can provide, you simply shouldn't eat or drink anything that has calories.

On the other hand, we also argue that small amounts of good fats will not hinder your goals if you are only looking to control your insulin.

And finally, we also say that some authors defend the idea that eating very few calories (up to 50 kcal) would not break your fast, regardless of the source of those calories.

Even so, we know that some people prefer a summary list of foods to help them get started.

This practical list helps to remember which foods and drinks can or cannot be consumed during the fast window, without necessarily "breaking your fast" or ending all its benefits.

126

For this reason, we have put down a short, non-exhaustive list of foods that can be eaten without disturbing your fast.

Question # 4:   But what about Sweetened Foods but No Calories? Like Coffee with Stevia, Erythritol or Sucralose, and even Zero Soda?

By now, you have understood that the idea of intermittent fasting is not to consume food, so as not to ingest calories, or to raise insulin.

So, using non-caloric sweeteners would be released, right?

Calm down, this issue is more complex than it may seem at first.

First, I strongly recommend that you understand the differences between the different types of low-carb sweeteners.

But, as we explained, even if we consider only sweeteners that do not raise insulin (as is the case with stevia, or even erythritol, for example), we still have an important question.

That (although this relationship is speculative, that is, unproven), there are possibly several potential mechanisms through which the use of sweeteners can interfere with metabolism.

And that even includes interactions with sweet taste receptors, which would stimulate other metabolic adaptations.

Certainly, more research is needed, but in our opinion, this is yet another sign that it can be smart not to abuse sweeteners.

And in our personal opinion, one thing is certain: the daily consumption of sweeteners is not ideal for your health, even though it may not hinder weight loss or break your fast.

Especially in the case of artificial sweeteners, and even more so in the case of zero soft drinks.

Question # 5:   Who Can Do Intermittent Fasting?

An important question that people often have when we talk about fasting and its benefits is precisely who can and cannot fast (practice it).

The direct answer is that the practice of intermittent fasting is suitable for healthy adults.

It is even easier to speak who should not start fasting without first talking to their trusted doctor.

Question # 6:   But Isn't Eating Right every 3 Hours?

Not really.

As we explained in our text, "Eat every 3 hours," "Do you still fall for that lie?" "People adopt this practice for 4 alleged reasons."

That is, they think that eating every 3 hours will help them:

128

1. Speed up the metabolism.
2. Control blood glucose.
3. Control appetite.
4. Preserve your muscle mass.

However, these 4 points are controversial (not to say wrong) in the light of science, and eating every few hours may even make some of these results worse.

Again, if you want a more detailed explanation on this point, I recommend reading our full text on eating every 3 or 4 hours.

Question # 7:   Does Fasting Slow Metabolism?

If you are paying attention to this text, you should already intuitively know the answer to that question.

No, intermittent fasting does not slow down metabolism.

The keyword in this sentence is "intermittent."

For it is clear that to spend very long periods (several and several days) without eating will imply a metabolic adaptation (that is, a slowing down of the metabolism).

Just as a very long and/or severe caloric restriction will also have the same effect.

This is because our body seeks to survive above all else.

So, if you go without eating for several days, your body will seek to preserve energy.

However, on short fasts, our metabolism tends to increase.

In this case, one study found a 3.6% increase in metabolism on short fasts, and another study found that metabolism increased 10% during fasting.

This makes evolutionary sense: if our body seeks to feed, it needs to stimulate us, and not deprive us of the energy we have, so that we can hunt/collect food and thus obtain energy.

This is probably mediated by hormonal changes that occur during fasting, such as increased adrenaline.

Question # 8:   Intermittent Fasting Causes Loss of Muscle Mass (Lean Mass)?

Another very common question is regarding the conservation of muscle mass when we practice fasting.

This question arises mainly because we always hear around (especially repeated as a mantra in gyms), that if you didn't eat every three hours, your body would start to burn muscles to provide you with energy.

Unfortunately, this is a very common myth, and we just have no idea where it came from.

130

If you read the question about "eating every 3 hours" that we answered above, then you understand that you don't have to eat every 3 hours to conserve your muscle mass.

On the other hand, you may be wondering if taking longer periods without eating (16, 24, 48 hours, or more) would damage your lean mass.

But you can rest easy: during the fasting window, you will not break muscles as a form of energy.

In fact, your muscles can even serve as an energy source, but you have other reserves that are much easier for your body to use, such as fat in your belly and elsewhere, and glycogen.

Remembering that glycogen is our energy reserve in the form of carbohydrates, which is stored both in the liver and in the muscles, between the muscle cells.

Question # 9:   Can I Exercise during Fasting?

Another very common question concerns fasting and physical exercise.

The most common questions are:

1. Can I train fasting?
2. Can I not eat anything after training?
3. Can I train fasting and continue fasting afterward?

Briefly, the answer to these questions and their variations is: you can do what you want.

You can train on a fast if you feel good, for example.

At the same time, there are people who are not feeling well, in which case they probably shouldn't be training fasting.

Of course, if you're on a high-carb, especially refined diet, eating every three hours; for a low-carb diet and still, start fasting and training hard, so it's normal that you don't feel well.

You need to give your body time to adapt to all these changes.

However, we believe that most people can, yes, train fasting after some time of adaptation, if they want to do so.

That is, there is nothing special about being fasting that prevents you from training.

You can even practice fasting and then fast for a few more hours until your lunch.

As we mentioned in the case of lean gains fasting, you don't necessarily need to have your first meal right before or right after your workout.

Question # 10: Which Supplements Do Not Break Intermittent Fasting?

Now, that you know you can train on an empty stomach, without eating anything before and nothing afterward, maybe your next question is precisely related to supplements.

As we have said before, theoretically, fasting is a period when you should not eat anything.

However, there are exceptions, as in the case of insulin fasting.

So, it is natural that doubts related to supplements arise as well.

Especially because there are supplements that do not really break the fast because they do not contain calories.

Question # 11: What to Say When Someone Criticizes your Fasting?

The truth is that, even with all the support that science gives to this practice, fasting is still a controversial topic for most people.

(As strange as, it may be that we live in a society in which we skip meals occasionally and eat real food are controversial.)

So, don't be alarmed if you receive unwanted criticism or comments from friends and family.

Conclusion

You have been given all the tools you might need, so as to learn all there is to know about intermittent fasting over the age of 50. Now it is all up to you. You should know by now how valuable this type of feeding rotation can be for you, especially as you are growing older. It is not just about shedding some extra pounds or boosting your metabolism. It is also about increasing your lifespan, making you feel healthier and more content about things that happen every day. This is a once-in-a-lifetime opportunity to reset your body and literally start over. Don't you want this transformation?

This is just the beginning of the journey. You might feel anxious, a little overwhelmed by information, and eager to see what lies ahead. Don't be in a hurry. Let the journey take you where you want to be, offering you amazing benefits throughout the whole process. After all, it is a work in progress. As you dive deeper, you get to realize more details about intermittent fasting. You discover more things about the way your own body works and responds to different situations. Over time, you comprehend which foods are good for you and which ones you should omit from your diet plan. And as you are seeing that transformation slowly taking place, your determination becomes stronger. It is fascinating, learning to interpret the signs and allowing your body to heal itself.

Do not just choose to fast, without first reading all about it. This would be a disaster. You should know by now your body is complex, with various layers in need of exploration. So, give yourself some time to study and realize what is best for you in the long run. Turn to science, whenever you are experiencing even the slightest sliver of doubt. Do not let it simmer, as it is going to grow into an even more important issue over time. Clear the air, let nothing unanswered; and when you are ready, ease yourself into the process of intermittent fasting.

I hope this book has been inspirational in your journey, which is about to start now. I am wishing you all the best, and I am looking forward to the revolutionary changes which are about to take place in your life. It is an exciting thing to see people who have chosen intermittent fasting, as they are changing from within. They look radiant, totally transformed, and filled with hope for the future.